CREATING A BUSINESS CASE FOR QUALITY IMPROVEMENT RESEARCH

EXPERT VIEWS

WORKSHOP SUMMARY

Samantha Chao, *Rapporteur*

Forum on the Science of Health Care Quality
Improvement and Implementation

Board on Health Care Services

INSTITUTE OF MEDICINE
OF THE NATIONAL ACADEMIES

THE NATIONAL ACADEMIES PRESS
Washington, D.C.
www.nap.edu

THE NATIONAL ACADEMIES PRESS   500 Fifth Street, N.W.   Washington, DC 20001

NOTICE: The project that is the subject of this report was approved by the Governing Board of the National Research Council, whose members are drawn from the councils of the National Academy of Sciences, the National Academy of Engineering, and the Institute of Medicine.

This project was supported by a grant from the Robert Wood Johnson Foundation and Award No. HHSP233200700506P between the National Academy of Sciences and the Department of Health and Human Services. Any opinions, findings, conclusions, or recommendations expressed in this publication are those of the author(s) and do not necessarily reflect the view of the organizations or agencies that provided support for this project.

International Standard Book Number-13:   978-0-309-11652-7
International Standard Book Number-10:   0-309-11652-X

Additional copies of this report are available from the National Academies Press, 500 Fifth Street, N.W., Lockbox 285, Washington, DC 20055; (800) 624-6242 or (202) 334-3313 (in the Washington metropolitan area); Internet, http://www.nap.edu.

For more information about the Institute of Medicine, visit the IOM home page at: www.iom.edu.

The serpent has been a symbol of long life, healing, and knowledge among almost all cultures and religions since the beginning of recorded history. The serpent adopted as a logotype by the Institute of Medicine is a relief carving from ancient Greece, now held by the Staatliche Museen in Berlin.

IOM (Institute of Medicine). 2008. *Creating a business case for quality improvement research: Expert views, workshop summary.* Washington, DC: The National Academies Press.

"Knowing is not enough; we must apply.
Willing is not enough; we must do."
—Goethe

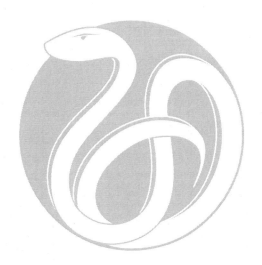

INSTITUTE OF MEDICINE
OF THE NATIONAL ACADEMIES

Advising the Nation. Improving Health.

THE NATIONAL ACADEMIES
Advisers to the Nation on Science, Engineering, and Medicine

The **National Academy of Sciences** is a private, nonprofit, self-perpetuating society of distinguished scholars engaged in scientific and engineering research, dedicated to the furtherance of science and technology and to their use for the general welfare. Upon the authority of the charter granted to it by the Congress in 1863, the Academy has a mandate that requires it to advise the federal government on scientific and technical matters. Dr. Ralph J. Cicerone is president of the National Academy of Sciences.

The **National Academy of Engineering** was established in 1964, under the charter of the National Academy of Sciences, as a parallel organization of outstanding engineers. It is autonomous in its administration and in the selection of its members, sharing with the National Academy of Sciences the responsibility for advising the federal government. The National Academy of Engineering also sponsors engineering programs aimed at meeting national needs, encourages education and research, and recognizes the superior achievements of engineers. Dr. Charles M. Vest is president of the National Academy of Engineering.

The **Institute of Medicine** was established in 1970 by the National Academy of Sciences to secure the services of eminent members of appropriate professions in the examination of policy matters pertaining to the health of the public. The Institute acts under the responsibility given to the National Academy of Sciences by its congressional charter to be an adviser to the federal government and, upon its own initiative, to identify issues of medical care, research, and education. Dr. Harvey V. Fineberg is president of the Institute of Medicine.

The **National Research Council** was organized by the National Academy of Sciences in 1916 to associate the broad community of science and technology with the Academy's purposes of furthering knowledge and advising the federal government. Functioning in accordance with general policies determined by the Academy, the Council has become the principal operating agency of both the National Academy of Sciences and the National Academy of Engineering in providing services to the government, the public, and the scientific and engineering communities. The Council is administered jointly by both Academies and the Institute of Medicine. Dr. Ralph J. Cicerone and Dr. Charles M. Vest are chair and vice chair, respectively, of the National Research Council.

www.national-academies.org

FORUM ON THE SCIENCE OF HEALTH CARE QUALITY IMPROVEMENT AND IMPLEMENTATION

THOMAS F. BOAT (*Co-Chair*), Department of Pediatrics, University of Cincinnati College of Medicine

PAUL H. O'NEILL (*Co-Chair*), Former U.S. Secretary of the Treasury, Pittsburgh, PA

PAUL B. BATALDEN, Director, Health Care Improvement Leadership Development, Dartmouth Medical School, Hanover, NH

IGNATIUS BAU, Program Director, The California Endowment, San Francisco, CA

JAY E. BERKELHAMER, Senior Vice President of Medical Affairs, Children's Healthcare of Atlanta

MARSHALL H. CHIN, Associate Professor of Medicine and Co-Director, General Internal Medicine Research, University of Chicago

CAROLYN M. CLANCY,* Director, Agency for Healthcare Research and Quality, Rockville, MD

CATHERINE D. DEANGELIS, Editor-in-Chief, *Journal of the American Medical Association* Scientific Publications and Multimedia Applications, Chicago, IL

JULIE L. GERBERDING,* Director, Centers for Disease Control and Prevention, Atlanta, GA

JEREMY GRIMSHAW, Director, Clinical Epidemiology Program, Ottawa Health Research Institute, Ontario, Canada

JEROME H. GROSSMAN, Senior Fellow, John F. Kennedy School of Government, Harvard University, Cambridge, MA

JUDITH GUERON, Scholar-in-Residence, MDRC, New York

ANDREA KABCENELL, Executive Director for Pursuing Perfection, Institute for Healthcare Improvement, Cambridge, MA

RICHARD KAHN, Chief Scientific and Medical Officer, American Diabetes Association, Alexandria, VA

RAYNARD S. KINGTON,* Deputy Director, Office of the Director, National Institutes of Health, Bethesda, MD

JOEL KUPERSMITH,* Chief Research and Development Officer, Veterans Health Administration, Washington, DC

LAURA C. LEVITON, Special Advisor for Evaluation, The Robert Wood Johnson Foundation, Princeton, NJ

BRIAN S. MITTMAN, Co-Editor-in-Chief, *Implementation Science*, and VA Greater Los Angeles Healthcare System, Sepulveda, CA

---

*Denotes ex-officio members.

STEPHEN M. SHORTELL, Blue Cross of California Distinguished Professor of Health Policy and Management, University of California, Berkeley

MARITA G. TITLER, Director, Institute for Translational Practice, University of Iowa City Health Care System and University of Iowa, Department of Nursing Services and Patient Care, Iowa City

KERRY WEEMS,[*] Acting Administrator, Centers for Medicare & Medicaid Services, Washington, DC

IOM Forum Staff

SAMANTHA CHAO, Forum Director
MICHELLE BAZEMORE, Senior Program Assistant[1]
CASSANDRA CACACE, Senior Program Assistant
ROGER HERDMAN, Board Director, Board on Health Care Services
MICHELE ORZA, Acting Board Director, Board on Health Care Services[1]

---

[1]Served through November 2007.

Reviewers

This report has been reviewed in draft form by individuals chosen for their diverse perspectives and technical expertise, in accordance with procedures approved by the National Research Council's Report Review Committee. The purpose of this independent review is to provide candid and critical comments that will assist the institution in making its published report as sound as possible and to ensure that the report meets institutional standards for objectivity, evidence, and responsiveness to the study charge. The review comments and draft manuscript remain confidential to protect the integrity of the deliberative process. We wish to thank the following individuals for their review of this report:

DONALD GOLDMANN, Institute for Healthcare Improvement, Cambridge, MA

STUART GUTERMAN, Program on Medicare's Future, The Commonwealth Fund, Washington, DC

SCOTT J. HAMLIN, Cincinnati Children's Hospital Medical Center, Cincinnati, OH

LAURA C. LEVITON, The Robert Wood Johnson Foundation, Princeton, NJ

SUSAN C. ROSSI, Office of Medical Applications of Research, National Institutes of Health, Bethesda, MD

Although the reviewers listed above have provided many constructive comments and suggestions, they were not asked to endorse the final draft of the report before its release. The review of this report was overseen by coordinator **DONALD M. STEINWACHS,** of Health Services Research and Development Center, Bloomberg School of Public Health, Johns Hopkins University. Appointed by the Institute of Medicine, he was responsible for making certain that an independent examination of this report was carried out in accordance with institutional procedures and that all review comments were carefully considered. Responsibility for the final content of this report rests entirely with the authoring committee and the institution.

in memoriam

This workshop summary is dedicated to
Dr. Jerome Grossman,
a pioneer in health informatics and health care quality,
a valued member of the forum,
and an irreplaceable colleague and friend.

Contents

Overview[*]

The Institute of Medicine (IOM) convened the workshop "Creating a Business Case for Quality Improvement and Quality Improvement Research" on October 15, 2007, in Washington, DC, to develop a better understanding of the economic and business disciplines that encourage sustained efforts to improve the quality of health care.

Throughout the country, institutional reluctance to invest in quality improvement and documentation of outcomes of quality improvement interventions remains a barrier to moving ahead, said Thomas Boat, co-chair of the Forum on the Science of Health Care Quality Improvement and Implementation. This reluctance stems from limited resources and, more importantly, competing priorities as to how these resources are spent within health care. For example, priorities tend to be placed on creating highly visible technology-driven programs, with less emphasis on meeting the needs and expectations of patients. Articulating a business case[1] is

---

[*]The planning committee's role was limited to planning the workshop. The workshop summary has been prepared by the workshop rapporteur as a factual summary of what occurred at the workshop.

[1]The following is a generally accepted definition of the business case but was not discussed or adopted during the workshop or by the planning committee. "A business case for a health care improvement intervention exists if the entity that invests in the intervention realizes a financial return on its investment in a reasonable time

at the crux of the issue of how rapidly quality improvement and quality improvement research will advance, Boat said.

The United States health care system is currently being threatened because it is not performing optimally, said Scott Hamlin, leader of the planning committee for the workshop. In every other industry, quality has been recognized as a necessity for value. We must understand what it is about health care that causes skepticism about whether the health care market can recognize quality and the rewards it brings so that we can capitalize on opportunities to strengthen the health care system.

During this workshop, experts were asked to discuss the business case from the perspectives of those actually making the business case, policy makers, and researchers. The planning committee's statement of task for developing the workshop agenda was "to provide the forum with insight into the economic, public policy, and business disciplines that create a sustainable value proposition for aggressively pursuing quality improvement in the health care system and thereby stimulating meaningful research in this field."

In summary, speakers indicated that a business case for quality improvement can indeed be made. Many examples of business cases from a variety of settings were provided, while recognizing that robust research is at the core of the business case for quality improvement. A strong research base and data depicting the impact of quality improvement are necessary to create a business case for quality improvement.

Throughout the workshop, common themes emerged. Making the right thing to do through systems change and leadership were recognized as necessary to improve quality of care delivery. Data and data transparency are also important for making health care more patient-centric. Speakers addressed funding as a key component of quality improvement and research on quality improvement due to the need to support the incorporation of health care innovations into practice. During the workshop, it was also noted that training must be enhanced to make research on quality improvement more robust. Finally, speakers discussed how the quality improvement and research communities must become better communicators and

---

frame, using a reasonable rate of discounting. This may be realized as bankable dollars (profit), a reduction in losses for a given program or population, or avoided costs. In addition, a business case may exist if the investing entity believes that a positive indirect effect on organizational function and sustainability will accrue within a reasonable time frame" (Leatherman et al., 2003).

include chief executive officers and chief financial officers, as well as patients and their families, in the ongoing dialogue to improve health care.

The following chapters describe and summarize workshop presentations and discussions. Therefore, the content is limited to the views presented and discussed during the workshop itself and is not intended to be a comprehensive assessment of the business case for health care quality improvement. The broader scope of issues pertaining to this subject area is recognized but could not be addressed in this summary. Appendix A is the workshop agenda, and Appendix B lists workshop participants.

The forum is used by the IOM to convene representatives from academia, government, and industry. In bringing together this broad group of stakeholders with diverse views, the forum provides a neutral setting where issues related to improving the science supporting health care quality improvement and implementation can be discussed. Through their discussions, forum members attain a better understanding of what the needs are and begin crossing the communication barriers that prevent advances in the field.

1

The Business Case for Quality Improvement

"Value—Not everything that can be counted counts, and not everything that counts can be counted."

—Einstein

The workshop convened a panel of five practitioners and managers to learn about different views of the business cases that have been made in health care. Although each speaker comes from a different background, there is a need to think about how each view contributes to the creation of a high-value health care system for the general population, said Paul O'Neill, forum co-chair. Speakers were asked to address at least two of the following questions:

- Is there a business case in today's health care environment that is responsive and relevant to the leadership of health care and related research enterprises (including providers, payers, patients, government officials, academia, and employers)?
- If so, what are the economic/financial benefits of pursuing quality improvements and related research in the field? Illustrate how quality improvement and quality improvement research can impact greater production use of plant and human assets, lead to product differentiation and branding, generate revenue enhancements, improve cost structure, and impact other core operational goals to create competitive advantages.
- What are the characteristics of an ideal enterprise culture and effective governance orientation that promote and accelerate improvement in quality and quality improvement research?
- What are the business disciplines and support structures that are essential for leadership to fully exploit the economic/

financial benefits of quality improvement and quality improvement research?

• In order to drive organizational improvement from validated, well-researched data, how do you effectively measure and evaluate progress against quality improvement targets and quantify returns on investments made? What are the essential components of such a system?

• Are there models in other industries such as aviation and nuclear power wherein the drive for quality has transformed product outcomes and customer/public safety? How do we learn from them?

MANAGED CARE

Herb Fritch of HealthSpring, a managed care company, engages physicians in making a business case for quality improvement as part of HealthSpring's business plan. HealthSpring, located in six states, specializes in Medicare Advantage plans that cover 150,000 lives and yields $1.5 billion in annual revenue. HealthSpring considers its physicians to be key elements of costs, outcomes, and quality. Part of its responsibility is to help organize large networks of independent physicians in which physicians themselves create risk-sharing structures.

Fritch described HealthSpring's pay-for-quality program, which focuses on ensuring that preventive care and chronic disease management are based on evidence (as measured by 25 measures of quality and outcomes) for small groups of providers. According to Fritch, 15 percent to 50 percent of physician reimbursement should ideally be linked to performance, measured in terms of cost, quality, and outcomes. This requires collection of data at the individual physician level (e.g., resource use and outcomes), governance, and clinical support. In a pilot program, HealthSpring provided physicians with support services, such as nurses, to improve care delivery. In a physician group provided with support services, Fritch saw a 20 percent to 25 percent improvement in performance, as well as a 5 percent decrease in costs from the initial state. Specifically, support services and a focus on primary care for chronic disease management have resulted in improved care, fewer emergency room visits, and fewer admissions, yielding large financial savings. Costs actually increased 5 percent to 10 percent among HealthSpring's other providers. With this success, HealthSpring decided to expand the program to four other markets; in 2006 it served eight groups, or approximately 9,000 patients. In 2007 the program expanded to

31 groups, or approximately 27,000 patients and 330 primary care physicians.

HealthSpring's pay-for-quality program costs an average of $10 extra per member per month, which includes the costs associated with support persons, program expenses, and physician bonuses. The estimated savings from fewer admissions and better health outcomes were approximately $45 per member per month, Fritch said. Many indirect nonmonetary benefits were also associated with the programs, such as better relationships between HealthSpring and physicians due to the potential for bonuses (which may be awarded three to four times a year) and the support services provided. Additionally, the ability to help organize primary care physicians facilitated HealthSpring's efforts to develop incentives for efficiency.

In its path to a successful pay-for-quality program, HealthSpring identified many challenges. Although its program worked in a Medicare Advantage setting, it is unclear whether this pay-for-quality program would easily translate to a fee-for-service setting. The program worked in a managed care, capitated payment system because the care was focused on primary care services and referrals. Primary care physicians therefore often followed their patients across the entire spectrum of health care services and had access to all of their health information, becoming a patient's "medical home." Patients were happier with the care they received because the care was more patient centered, as best shown in settings offering concierge services, such as HealthSpring's Personal Assistant Liaison program, which provides one-on-one support to help members manage their own care.

One critical factor in HealthSpring's success was the addition of electronic medical records to promote evidence-based medicine. However, benefits of electronic records were seen in some clinical areas, but not others. For patients seen in fee-for-service payment systems, the use of electronic records required an extra 30 seconds to treat each patient, which was not sustainable across a volume of 40 patients per day per physician. Instead, savings were derived largely by providing evidence-based care for expensive services, such as managing chronic diseases. If the program was to be generalized to a fee-for-service system, the major stakeholder, Medicare, must become the driver of change, Fritch said.

DEPARTMENT OF VETERANS AFFAIRS

Information is extremely important in driving change because it indicates when a problem exists, said James Bagian of the Department of Veterans Affairs (VA). From his perspective as director of patient safety at the VA, Bagian believes the data show that a business case for quality improvement exists. For every $100 spent on VA operations, 10 cents is spent on implementing patient safety programs, equating to $130,000 per facility per year. The cost of adverse events is much greater, exemplified by the following:

- Falls resulting in fractures cost an average of $25,000 to $35,000 per fracture (more importantly, one in three patients over age 65 with a fall-related fracture dies).
  - Adverse drug events cost approximately $5,000 per event.
  - Nosocomial infections cost a minimum of $5,000 per episode.

These costs, aggregated from data outside the VA, resulted in losses for the institutions where the adverse events occurred. In terms of benefit ratios, Bagian provided the following data on savings:

- An investment of $1,000 in hand hygiene yielded $60,000 in avoided care costs.
- An investment of $25,000 in a fall prevention program yielded $115,000 in savings in fracture care.

Chief executive officers (CEOs) and chief financial officers (CFOs) often express strong resistance to changes in care until cost–benefit analyses are provided, Bagian said. With the data, the benefits of quality improvement quickly become apparent.

The need to create a business case for quality improvement is only one constraint to providing high-value health care; it is not the goal. The ultimate goal of health care is to improve patient care and safety, while the ultimate goal of patient safety is to prevent inadvertent harm to the patient resulting from the care he or she receives. But who should ultimately be responsible for quality and patient safety? In a survey taken within the Veterans Health Administration (part of the VA) and other private health care organizations, only 27 percent of respondents believed patient safety was important for good patient care. Yet safety should be everyone's concern, Bagian said. No health care provider or institution is immune. The culture of health care is a driving force behind the health care problem because health care providers are plagued by both ignorance (i.e., trying to be perfect, an impossible goal, instead of recognizing the role that common system failures play in causing harm) and arrogance (i.e., believing the problem lies with everyone else). As a cultural issue, quality has not been well understood. Medicine has been viewed more as a cottage industry in which practice is either based on physicians' personal preferences or unsubstantiated by evidence. With a lack of standardization and accountability, medicine has not been viewed as an effective, efficient system.

Bagian suggested that the way in which medicine is organized needs to be redesigned to induce change. In medicine, there is little understanding of how systems function in relation to people and processes. Not enough people in health care even know what systems-based solutions would look like because most health care professionals are not trained in systems engineering, Bagian said, although this concept is starting to be incorporated into some parts of medicine (e.g., Accreditation Council for Graduate Medical Education). From a systems approach, Bagian suggested that current interventions are aimed at the wrong level: The primary focus should be on changing systems, not on correcting individual physicians.

Other industries have achieved change. Bagian described lessons learned from aviation in World War I, where 14,000 Royal Air Force pilots were killed, 8,000 of whom were killed during training. A similar situation occurred in the United States during World War II; as more planes crashed, more were built, and pilots were replaced. This continued until Congress decided it could no longer support such a system. The military was forced to develop programs and to find opportunities within the system to minimize accidents. In 1954 the United States Navy destroyed 774 aircraft. The implementation of standardized systems resulted in dramatic reductions in mishaps; in 1996 only 39 aircraft were destroyed. If a process deviated from the norm, a reason had to be given. People finally began to understand the value of using procedures and checklists to reduce mistakes.

Change requires goals, which must be clear, compelling, and reinforced by leadership. Change in health care is not just about reducing costs; it is more about improving value and delivering good care. This must be understood to enlist the support of care providers. The goal must be clearly articulated by leadership, so that various ways to achieve the goal can be developed.

Many obstacles prevent systems change. One obstacle is problem recognition. Many health care professionals believe their level of performance is above average, so statements about substandard performance do not apply. Good data systems are needed to show physicians their actual levels of performance and how they compare to others so improvement efforts can be strategically targeted. A second obstacle is fear of punishment, blame, and the shame in having made mistakes. The current system does not encourage reporting of mistakes, but instead fuels a culture of hiding errors, which precludes learning from other people's mistakes. Fear is also the cost of implementing safer systems. A third obstacle to systems change occurs when mistakes are made and people do not know what to do because adequate systems are not in place to change the way they practice. A fourth obstacle is a lack of evidence showing that different practices or tools can improve care. This type of evidence can galvanize behavioral and attitudinal change, steps necessary for cultural change.

One tool used by the VA to change culture focused on removing workers' fear of making mistakes, introduced as the concept of blameworthiness. It was well known that issues associated with health professionals involved in criminal acts, substance abuse, or intentionally unsafe acts would become public, and punishment would follow. However, by changing the environment and clarifying that only those types of activities were subject to punitive measures, workers reporting unintentional errors to the safety system could feel safe. The VA experienced a 30-fold increase in reporting in the first year; this rate has increased continuously over the past 8 years, Bagian said. For the concept of blameworthiness to succeed, the program needed to be fair and transparent, requiring the VA to develop precise definitions with unions, patient groups, and oversight committees before the program was initiated. The confidentiality of error reporting was another critical factor for success. It ensured that the name of the reporter was never revealed, except in cases of criminal acts, substance abuse, or intentionally unsafe acts, as different systems exist to deal with those cases. Quality and safety programs should not be mixed with accountability systems, Bagian argued.

The criteria for prioritizing errors must be made transparent for both internal and external purposes. The VA developed a single set of prioritization criteria based on risk—defined as both severity and probability of an event's occurrence—that was used to satisfy multiple regulatory bodies, such as the Food and Drug Administration, the Joint Commission, and the Centers for Disease Control and Prevention (CDC). This set of criteria made it procedurally easier to meet requirements of all regulatory bodies and allowed for greater transparency to patients, professional organizations, and other external stakeholders.

Human error is not a cause of error, but rather an effect of systems error. If human error is the cause, the solution is to avoid mistakes. The more practical solution is to change the system so that making mistakes is difficult, Bagian explained. For example, potassium chloride, a potentially fatal chemical compound, was once available in concentrated form on hospital floors. Now it is premixed in intravenous bags to avoid errors. Management must be involved in safety efforts by talking about it and making it a priority and a regular part of all activities; it is a marathon, not a sprint. Identifying causes of errors requires root cause analyses, but solving errors requires development of actions, outcome measures, and a commitment to provide resources necessary for change. If the resources cannot be committed, a new action plan must be developed to fit within those constraints. The process and rationale for this decision-making process must be communicated clearly between management and frontline personnel.

The focus of research must be different, Bagian explained. Evaluation of actions is critical, both in terms of processes and outcomes. One example is physician hand hygiene. The effect of hand washing on infection rates has been shown and does not need to be studied again; however, research should be conducted to examine whether physicians actually wash their hands properly and the factors associated with the obstacles to achieving success. The following elements are necessary for sustainable improvement:

- Appropriate goal identification and selection
- Transparent prioritization
- Identification of real causes
- System-based countermeasures that address underlying causes
- Explicit, strong actions
- Measurement of actions
- Top leadership involvement/visibility

Research on how to get people to do the right thing is needed, Bagian asserted. Some research has been completed determining what the right thing to do is, but implementing the right thing is much more complicated.

SYSTEMS

Toward the end of marathons, there tends to be a gap between the leaders and the other runners, said Steve Spear of the Institute for Healthcare Improvement and the Massachusetts Institute of Technology. The leaders run with effortless strides and composed faces. They are followed by a second group of runners who are still impressive, but not quite as composed; this pattern of decline continues through the rest of the groups of marathon runners. What is the difference between the leaders and the rest of the pack? The runners all have similar access to training facilities and nutrition, but front runners always emerge, Spear said. Applying this analogy to industries, how does a company become the pacesetter within its own industry? Competing companies work within the same regulations, develop similar products in similar sectors, and work with the same customers, suppliers, and worker pools. The competition should be cutthroat, but consistent leaders exist for a variety of industries, with pacesetters' market caps and profitability being far greater than those of the rest of the industry (e.g., leaders such as Toyota, Alcoa, and Southwest Airlines).

The implication for health care, Spear stated, is that great science offers hope for improvement. There is a lot of hope that care can improve and costs can decrease, but performance is poor because there is a gap between promise and delivery. Twenty to 50 years ago, medical science was in its infancy. Breast cancer, for example, was thought of as one disease. It is now known that the term "breast cancer" is actually an umbrella term for dozens of types of cancers. This evolution in thinking came as a result of better science, which gives hope for advancement. In 1955 a physician managing the care of a patient with breast cancer either provided mostly palliative care or performed radical mastectomies in hopes of a cure. Both require the management of small teams (e.g., surgical team and postoperative team). The bad news was that the science was poor, causing teams to practice and advance disciplines within silos. The good news was that patients were being treated in a simple system where the difficulty of coordination between teams did not have to be faced.

That situation has now changed. The good news is that the science has improved dramatically. The bad news, however, is that scientific advances require deep knowledge of specific issues, so as science advances, what one person knows becomes more and more narrow. This makes the task of managing the care of all patients going through a system nearly impossible for one person. Each patient is individualized, making systems failures difficult to identify. Physicians are now practicing in a complex system. Physicians struggle to balance constantly advancing science with the interdependencies and unknown interactions between complex systems. Coordination and collaboration must become the focus of systems, Spear said.

The underperformance of health care is often noted, Spear said. This is not because the individual fails, as Bagian also recognized; individuals often perform extraordinarily well. *The system is what fails.* One reason systems fail is that they are managed in pieces when the focus should be on managing the integration of the pieces. The

---

BOX 1-1
An Example of System Failure

A woman recovering from a successful elective surgery suffered full-body seizures. No tests could explain the symptoms. When she returned to the nursing unit, it was discovered that she had low glucose levels, but the discovery came too late and the patient died.

Heparin, a blood thinner, is a clear, colorless liquid, stored in a glass vial. The night nurse had responded to an alarm to break a blood clot and instead had inadvertently administered insulin. Insulin is also a clear, colorless liquid and contained in vials of about the same size, shape, and weight as the heparin vials. The print labeling on both vials was tiny and hard to read in the dark. The nurse inadvertently administered insulin as opposed to heparin, which caused the death of the patient.

Should the nurse be at fault? Should the pharmacy be at fault? No, because although the work of the pharmacy was good from its own perspective, it was bad from the perspective of the nurse. In fact, the system was at fault because of the lack of understanding of the interaction *between* the elements: the actual administration of the medication.

---

current system makes it too easy to do the wrong thing, explained Spear. The system must change to make it easy to do the right thing. As Box 1-1 indicates, there is a need to measure outcomes, not of individual actions, but of how well the parts of the system work together.

To prevent breakdowns within systems, Spear offered two solutions. First, people currently work in silos, leaving no manager of patient care from start to finish. People need to be held responsible for processes within organizations to complement what is already going on in care facilities. Second, the system needs to change so that the behavior of catching and reporting mistakes is rewarded. Mistakes and problems are solved only when they are elevated. The system needs to be managed as a whole, not in pieces; when problems are identified, they must be dealt with in order to achieve a safer health care system.

INTEGRATED HEALTH CARE SYSTEM

The journey to high-quality, efficient systems is a long one, said Gary Kaplan, CEO of the Virginia Mason Medical System. The journey is one of culture change. Virginia Mason's goal is to change in such a way that it may influence the ability to transform the health care industry. Virginia Mason is a not-for-profit integrated health care system with a 336-bed hospital and 480 physicians in 9 locations. Its vision is to be a leader in quality.

In describing Virginia Mason's strategic plan, Kaplan said the patient is the customer. But in 2001, processes and systems were designed around physicians, nurses, and other health givers, not the patient. To address this structure, Virginia Mason adopted the Virginia Mason Production System, modeled after the Toyota Production System, to deliver the best products and services possible to customers. Now in its sixth year of implementation, culture change has become the largest part of the strategy. A culture of feedback must be instilled, along with measures to ensure responsibility and accountability of both good and bad actions. People must be held accountable when lives are both saved and lost.

To enforce this culture change, Virginia Mason developed a compact with its physicians. Traditionally in group practices, compacts tend to mean physicians will be protected, have autonomy, and have a sense of entitlement, leading to a physician-centered health care environment, Kaplan said. However, in an environment focused on evidence-based guidelines and patient safety, the traditional compact is inappropriate, leading Virginia Mason to develop a new compact. This compact details the responsibilities of both the organization and its physicians. For example, one physician responsibility is to take ownership, including "implementing Virginia Mason–accepted clinical standards of care." These are best practices as shown by evidence and should be delivered to every patient every time unless there is a clear clinical rationale for not following the evidence-based best practice.

Quality has been defined by Virginia Mason with the following equation:

$$\text{Quality} = \text{Appropriateness} \times \frac{(\text{Outcomes} + \text{Service})}{\text{Waste}}$$

It was discovered that reducing waste on the non-value-added variations of services can improve quality and simultaneously reduce cost. In addition, if a procedure is performed correctly but is unnecessary, then there is no quality. Much of what is done in medicine is unnecessary and is done for a number of reasons, Kaplan said. At Virginia Mason, many processes have more than 50 percent waste. Examples from other industries are shown in Table 1-1.

To address the problem of waste, Virginia Mason turned to the

TABLE 1-1 Validated Industry Averages

Target	Percentage Reduction
Direct labor/productivity improved	45–75
Cost reduced	25–55
Throughput/flow increased	60–90
Quality (defects/scrap) reduced	50–90
Inventory reduced	60–90
Space reduced	35–50
Lead time reduced	50–90

NOTE: Summarized results, subsequent to a 5-year evaluation, from numerous companies (more than 15 aerospace related). Companies ranged from 1 to >7 years in lean principles application/execution.

Toyota Production System, the purpose of which is to standardize processes and remove waste to deliver what is needed, when it is needed, and where it is needed. A key to this is mistake proofing in real time, which has yielded better, faster, and more affordable products. Much of the stated opposition to standardization comes from the belief that people in such a system would be pushed toward widespread mediocrity; however, standardization is about widespread standard best practices, Kaplan explained. Double-blind control evidence supports only about one-third of health care delivered; the rest is emerging evidence. For care based on emerging evidence, standards should be set so this care can be measured and therefore be proven at the level of controlled studies. A lack of double-blind control evidence is often used as an excuse for variation, Kaplan stated. Instead, procedures for which there is no evidence should also be standardized to avoid error-prone situations.

In standardizing some of its processes, Virginia Mason discovered that much of the waste and delays could be condensed, reducing costs and time spent. When an insurer pointed out that Virginia Mason was not as cost-effective as it could be in certain areas, it looked for ways to make its processes more cost-effective. The company engaged in a process with the insurer, providers, and employers to focus on the highest cost diagnoses and applied evidence-based guidelines, with lean and cost accounting to redesign care delivery. This is exemplified by the back pain "value stream," depicted in Figure 1-1. Before the processes were streamlined, patients with back pain waited a long time for appointments with a primary care physician, referrals to magnetic resonance imaging (MRI), and neurosurgery. After applying the Virginia Mason Production System,

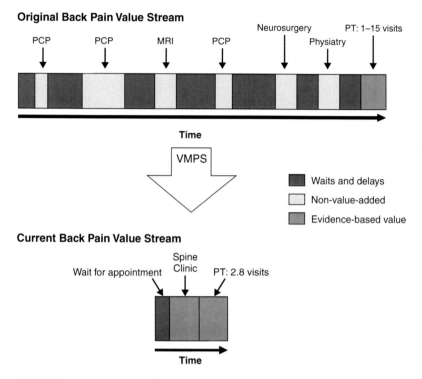

FIGURE 1-1 Back pain value streams.
NOTE: PCP = primary care physician; MRI = magnetic resonance imaging; PT = physical therapy; VMPS = Virginia Mason Production System.

changes were made to the system that reduced that waiting period. For example, patients were able to be seen on the same day in the spine clinic. As a result, overall waiting time decreased from more than a month to one day; fewer patients received MRIs due to more specific decision rules about who should receive MRIs; and patient satisfaction improved as patients were able to return to work more quickly. With this process, a business case for quality was also made. For back pain, Virginia Mason originally made profits only on MRIs, but after standardizing processes and dramatically reducing numbers of MRIs, the employer agreed to triple payments for physical therapy to allow Virginia Mason to break even. The revised, more efficient processes required fewer staff and saved the employer $17 per hour in indirect costs.

Due to its success, the Virginia Mason Production System has been used to improve processes when a number of other diagnoses arise (e.g., migraines, irregular heart rhythm, heartburn). This has led to a decrease in use of services, especially emergency room use and MRI use. The cumulative savings from 2005 to 2006 from decreased use of the emergency room and MRI totaled around $7.8 million.

Kaplan shared some lessons from his experiences. First, the Virginia Mason Production System has improved quality, access, and patient satisfaction and has decreased costs. This has led to an overall improvement in the value of care, leading Virginia Mason leaders to conclude that about half of health care costs may be avoidable. Another lesson was that the current payment system separates buyers and sellers. As alluded to in the back pain example, streamlining processes throughout the organization would be unsustainable if implemented broadly, for the organization would not be able to generate enough revenue. Therefore, payers must be enlightened enough to change the way they pay in fee-for-service payment systems and work with employers and providers. Aligning reimbursement with value is critical.

Culture change is a requirement for a higher quality delivery system. Leaders in health care need to address both the technical and human dimensions of change, Kaplan said. The technical dimension is the Virginia Mason Production System. The human dimension includes a number of components. First, a critical mass must articulate the urgency with which change must be addressed. Second, leaders must evolve from being advocates for physicians to being sponsors of change. Third, a broad and deep commitment to a shared vision is needed. Fourth, a new compact that aligns with the shared vision needs to be adopted. These components must be completed together to achieve culture change. Patients must come first, and there must be a shared belief in delivering zero-defect care. There is enough money in the health care system, Kaplan said. The challenge is to use what is in the system more wisely by removing waste and changing mind-sets.

NURSING PERSPECTIVE

Marita Titler of the University of Iowa was asked to briefly discuss the business case for quality improvement from the nursing perspective. Employed mostly in hospitals, nurses are the largest group of health care service providers in the United States, with a growing body of evidence that shows nurses contribute a great deal to quality of care and patient outcomes. Titler shared a number of examples based on improvements in nursing that not only improved quality, but also avoided costs.

The first example of cost avoidance was a cluster randomized trial to improve acute pain management for older adults with hip fractures, Titler explained. This study, funded by the Agency for Healthcare Research and Quality, investigated a translating research into practice (TRIP) intervention that included strategies to address communication processes, education, audit and feedback, outreach by an advanced practice nurse, and modifications in organizational standards of practice for acute pain management and clinical documentation tools. Study outcomes included measures of nurse and physician adoption of evidence-based acute pain management practices and improvements in pain intensity of patients. Pain assessments and pharmacological treatment practices improved at a statistically significant level. Patients experienced more around-the-clock administration of opioids, experienced less pain intensity, and received more evidence-based acute pain management care than those in the comparison group. The net cost savings of patient care for those in the experimental group was $1,500 per patient less than those in the comparison group. The TRIP intervention resulted in improved management of acute pain and saved the hospitals money.

Titler offered a second example of cost avoidance through quality improvement programs—the implementation of an advanced practice nurse transition model of care. Care delivered in accordance with this model improved care coordination, resulting in fewer readmissions, reduced numbers of hospital days, and increased percentages of patients without rehospitalizations. The net savings of the advanced practice nurse transition care model totaled $5,000 per patient and reduced total costs by 38 percent (McCauley et al., 2006; Naylor et al., 2004).

Efforts have also been made by quality improvement and interdisciplinary teams to address patient falls, which cost more than $20 billion in direct health care costs annually, Titler said. A program using unit-based scorecards and fall prevention interventions to reduce fall rates helped decrease falls and subsequent injuries, saving $100,000. Interestingly, a trend was found that correlated more fall prevention activities performed in a day with more money saved (Titler et al., 2005).

Retention of nurses is another important factor to consider, Titler noted. The costs of training new employees range from $75,000 to $115,000 per new hire. Efforts must be made to improve nurse retention rates because nurses are critical to continuous improvements in care. The findings from these examples should be applied broadly to improve patient care, Titler stated, reminding the workshop attendees that changes in health care must be directed toward promoting provision of evidence-based care to treat patients and improve patient outcomes. Nurses have a central role to play in making these necessary changes.

DISCUSSION

An open discussion followed the panel's presentations. Forum members and audience members (from the public) asked the speakers questions. The following sections summarize the discussion session.

Roles of Other Care Providers

In response to a question regarding the roles of nurses, Kaplan stated that nurses are critical to the execution of health care delivery and are integrally involved in delivery teams, process improvement, and the front lines of care. Although nurses have systems training in their education, as noted by Titler, most health care providers lack that type of training, Kaplan said. All players must be engaged to creatively and comprehensively change the system.

Bagian added that quality improvement is not "physicians versus nurses"; instead, everyone, both clinical and nonclinical, plays important roles. Interdisciplinary work is needed. Efforts to face challenges brought about by changing culture therefore must address physicians, nurses, and all other health care professionals. Each professional must change his or her own practices and adapt training to meet the demands of a changing health care system and, more importantly, the patient.

The role of incentives was discussed next. Incentives must be available for everyone in the system to produce a culture of safety, explained Bagian. People who report errors must receive some sort of incentive, which can be monetary or nonmonetary. Focusing on the nonmonetary incentives, Bagian said leadership is essential to creating honest and fair systems where problems can be fixed, motivating people to do the right things, and improving quality. Because safety is not just about financial rewards, good systems can motivate people to stay at institutions.

Fritch noted the high value that HealthSpring nurses add, especially in the care support and chronic disease management programs. One challenge is that bonuses provided by pay-for-performance programs are awarded to physicians who employ nurses, not the nurses actually doing the work. Some of HealthSpring's programs are now modifying their incentive programs to award to support staff and nurses.

Responding to the notion of nonmonetary incentives, Kaplan said that professional satisfaction is a key factor in reducing waste and work errors. For example, skill–task alignment should be considered so that nurses are not doing what technicians should be doing. There is a need to better understand value streams for all stages of work and to implement those findings to improve care.

Systems Change

Health care must be focused on the patient and how disciplines (e.g., physicians, nurses, occupational therapists) can collaborate to fix the care system to make it easy to do the right thing, Titler said.

Echoing Titler's point, health care professionals must share the belief that the purpose of health care is to provide good health care and improve or maintain the welfare of the public, Bagian said. Much progress has been made over the past decade, but change has been slow overall and not measurable in some places. If the system is to improve, the thinking cannot stay the same. First, a framework must articulate what needs to be accomplished to induce change (e.g., the goal of eliminating non-value-added care), followed by providing evidence for the framework, which together allow the system to reform. Payers of health care have to narrow down people's choices of health care providers so that only providers willing to provide high-quality, high-value care are rewarded. It must be broadly recognized that current resources are being misdirected.

Urgency for change does exist, Kaplan asserted. The system must tell and accept the truth. While some would say that Virginia Mason is different because it practices in community settings and an integrated system, the problems are the same: Evidence-based care is not followed consistently, and society is overpaying for medical procedures.

Advances made by Virginia Mason have been great, Fritch said, but cannot be widely implemented and sustained in the current health care system. Overall incentives need to change to encourage programs such as managed competition and capitated regional health systems so that health care organizations are not driven out of business by improving efficiency and eliminating waste.

Staff Competency

In response to a question about staff competency inhibiting quality improvement, Bagian suggested that the problem is more of a systems issue because not knowing how to assess competency or how to outline it is a management issue, not a personnel issue. For example, the vision of nurses and surgeons is seldom checked, if ever, but can be problematic and cause adverse events to occur. Instead of reacting only after an adverse event has occurred because of a vision limitation and dealing with a single practitioner, a more systems-based approach would mean that all individuals requiring a specific level of visual acuity be proactively evaluated.

Kaplan said that training and education are a big part of the problem. A lack of team-based training and systems training hinders progress. Simulation-based training could be used to ensure the competency of providers.

Bad systems can make the most competent people look incompetent, Spear said. In health care, it is often hard to find incompetent people, but it is very easy to find people who appear that way because the system often sabotages attempts to do the right thing. Physicians are poorly positioned to contribute to the well-being of systems because many never receive formal systems training. Additionally, physicians are not rewarded for the performance of the overall system, just their individual pieces.

Research

Pay for performance is producing results for only 50 percent to 55 percent of physicians, not 100 percent, which creates skepticism about whether financial incentives really can improve quality, Paul O'Neill said. Although a degree of patient compliance is involved, physician practices have the responsibility to implement improvement programs and change their own behaviors, responded Fritch. For example, one practice waived patient copays and provided the nurse support on its own.

When the CDC declared that beta blockers should be used in 90 percent of cardiac patients by 2010, the VA was already up to 99 percent, said Bagian. Some argue that the VA had such success because it is a military system, but this is false. The obstacles to care are much the same, and the realistic pressures of physician retention are the same. Physicians stay at the VA because of what they can do there, especially with the VA's electronic medical record. The patients are also involved through the electronic medical record.

Combined, these result in better systems of care, which allows the VA to perform well on those measures, Bagian explained.

Why more physicians do not participate in incentive programs is unclear, Fritch said. Some physicians do not believe the credibility of the data. Chart reviews have helped to allay some of the skepticism, but have not driven more people to change. This should be better understood.

Current measures of quality evaluate only discrete aspects of care, Bagian said. Measures tell people that something needs to be fixed, not how to fix it. The problem is that many providers do not know how to improve. Therefore, poor performance should not necessarily be deemed as ignorance on the part of providers. Research should be looking at and advancing processes of care, regardless of the process's utility. Often research can paralyze a process through analysis, Bagian argued.

The lack of systems integration and management must be researched, Spear said. Health care is now measured in many disciplines, but far less is captured about the experience of patients from start to finish. Drawing an analogy between health care and the automobile industry, the engine is not purchased from one place, the chassis from another, and the brakes from yet another. When consumers purchase cars, they let Toyota and General Motors worry about the integration. Yet, in health care, patients often manage the pieces and integrate them on their own. Additionally, consumer reports provide comparisons of different cars for people's different preferences. Learning about patient experiences in health care is not as easy. Processes must be measured to provide incentives to work on overall processes of care as opposed to specialties of care. Until that happens, it will be difficult for both payers and patients to make informed decisions, Spear said.

Transparency (and Consumers)

Transparency is about processes and measures, as well as the work, challenges, and foibles of doing better, Kaplan said. Only when the system is fully transparent can an environment conducive to high-performing teams of physicians, nurses, and others be created to reduce defects, improve value, and take inefficiencies out of the system. Although it is encouraging that some efforts have moved toward becoming more efficient, many people are resistant.

Agreeing with Kaplan, Bagian noted that transparency often is mentioned in the context of providing knowledge to consumers.

However, transparency is also critical internally within organizations, for people must feel comfortable acknowledging that they can harm patients, a mind-set that must be supported by organizational leadership. Fritch agreed, adding that consumers must be made aware of improved quality and have consistent access to such information.

2

The Role of Federal Funders

"Knowing is not enough; we must apply. Willing is not enough; we must do."

—Goethe

Policy makers recently have shown significant interest in trying to influence health care quality improvement, said Denise Cardo of the Centers for Disease Control and Prevention. The spectrum of policies varies widely among the federal, state, and, likely soon, consumer levels. The movement toward consumers is fueled by efforts to enhance transparency of outcomes and reimbursement policies. Although most policies are well intentioned, many are not evidence based. An opportunity therefore exists for evidence to improve implemented policies.

Panelists were asked by the planning committee to use the following questions as a guide for their remarks:

- What are the fundamental public policy features and objectives that will lead to a transformational improvement in the quality and economic viability of our health care system?
- What role does transparency of outcomes and cost data play in driving quality improvement? How can quality improvement research better support these efforts? What public policy features might help to unleash its potential?
- What public policy features are essential to help finance, promote, and reward relevant research into quality improvement sciences?

24

AGENCY FOR HEALTHCARE RESEARCH AND QUALITY

The federal government plays numerous roles in health care. It funds more than half of U.S. health care spending through various departments, such as the Department of Health and Human Services, the Department of Defense, and the Department of Veterans Affairs, said Carolyn Clancy of the Agency for Healthcare Research and Quality (AHRQ). Parts of the government are responsible for the actual provision of care, while others are responsible for informing health care decision makers. Although multiple factors influence health care quality and safety, policy initiatives must give organizations incentives to improve quality and share their experiences. Therefore, policy can be very helpful in shaping the environment in which care is delivered.

For the past decade, quality improvement has been a movement for health care leaders, but only recently has it become a movement for those on the front line of care delivery. In 2003 the Medicare Modernization Act required hospitals to report on selected measures of health care quality in order to receive their full reimbursements. Since then, the number of measures has grown, and beginning in 2008 hospitals will report on patient experiences of care through the Hospital CAHPS survey, Clancy said.

As recognized throughout the workshop, health care is a local enterprise. To build on this, Clancy introduced President Bush's four cornerstones of value-driven health care: (1) transparency of quality standards, (2) transparency of price standards, (3) information technology interoperability, and (4) incentives for providing high-quality care. To support the coordination of these cornerstones, regional and local public–private collaborations, or chartered value exchanges, have been developed. In support of this effort, AHRQ is developing a learning network to produce public reports, foster pay for performance, and thereby improve quality. Value exchanges will have some access to data at physician group levels, aggregated to distribute data on physician performance.

Evidence is used in making many types of policy decisions, from product approval to practice guidelines, from program financing to priority setting. But, Clancy asked, can a case be made for strengthening quality improvement research? The field is relatively new and the current evidence base is mixed about what works to improve quality, but it is becoming better understood that different research designs are needed for different methods. Randomized controlled trials are clearly helpful at times, but may not always be the best method. A large opportunity exists to use other methods, such as quasi-experimental methods. Context is also important to

capture, but it remains unclear how context should best be concep-
tualized and measured. If the connection between research on quality improvement and health care spending was better understood,
policy makers could do a lot to help build the science, Clancy said,
such as quickening the development of theories, better research
designs, and setting of priorities.

However, strengthening quality improvement research presents
many challenges. First, the ambiguous nature of quality makes it
difficult to understand. Second, the nature of funding for quality
improvement research poses a barrier. Third, the discovery of innovation almost always seems to be valued more than the use of
innovation, which may not be the correct view, Clancy said, for the
health care system cannot necessarily handle all health care innovations. To face these challenges, AHRQ is supporting a number of
activities, including programs such as the National Research Service
Awards, which focuses in part on funding quality improvement
research with explicit evaluation components for graduate and post-
doctoral research.

To garner more support for quality improvement research,
researchers must market the successes of individual quality improvement interventions. Conservative estimates of cost savings from
quality improvement (direct medical costs) exist (see Table 2-1), but
they are just the tip of the iceberg because they do not include avoidable sick days and other indirect costs, Clancy said. Communicat-

TABLE 2-1 Cost Savings from Quality Improvement

Topic	QI Focus	Cost Savings	Cost Type
Diabetes	Ambulatory care	$2.5 billion (2001)	Hospital costs
Hypertension	Ambulatory care	$292–$708 million	Hospital costs
Asthma (pediatric)	Ambulatory care	$600 million (2003)	Hospital costs
Waste	Efficiency	Up to $1 trillion	National health expenditures
Health care–associated infections	Hospital care	$5 billion (2000)	Hospital and other

NOTE: These cost savings can be found in the AHRQ *Closing the Quality Gap* series.
QI = quality improvement.

ing the economic benefits of interventions is not in the forefront of researchers' minds—a perspective that must change.

In changing the health care system, it cannot merely be insisted that changes be made; instead, actions must be taken, such as implementing smarter quality metrics as the basis for payment incentives so that the wrong behaviors are not rewarded up front. There is a need to understand more evidence-based management approaches, and to adjust policies to support them. We are just starting to look at the whole environment and need to become better at considering evidence and quality improvement research, Clancy said.

NATIONAL INSTITUTES OF HEALTH

The National Institutes of Health (NIH) is primarily a medical and behavioral research agency, not a health policy or health policy research agency, said Barnett Kramer of the NIH, voicing his personal opinions and not those of the federal agency. Although there is some overlap and support, quality improvement is not the main focus. As mentioned, there is a lack of coordination within the federal government regarding quality improvement in health care.

Paraphrasing the NIH mission statement, Kramer said the NIH's mission is science in the pursuit of fundamental knowledge about the nature and behavior of living systems and the application of that knowledge to extend healthy life and reduce the burdens of illness and disability. Many goals relate to achieving this mission, each with its own constituency and relevant budget. The primary focus of the NIH is the development of basic knowledge and interventions to improve health. Less focus exists on optimizing the delivery of those interventions, which some would categorize as health services. Quality improvement is an obvious yet relatively small component of a larger mission. However, a substantial amount of NIH-funded research informs quality of care, Kramer said. For example, research studying the efficacy of screenings for prostate cancer and new technologies provide data to determine whether these procedures should be implemented or whether the harms outweigh the benefits.

Health services research has constituted 3 percent of the NIH's annual budget, a percentage that has held relatively constant in the overall budget in recent years (see Table 2-2). The percentage of health services research that is devoted to quality improvement research is not specifically reported as a budget item. Of the 215 NIH study sections, only one focuses on health services and quality improvement: Health Services Organization and Delivery. This section reviews approximately 270 applications per year, largely

TABLE 2-2 Health Services Research as a Percentage of NIH Annual Budget by Fiscal Year (millions of dollars)

	FY 2003 (actual)	FY 2004 (actual)	FY 2005 (actual)	FY 2006 (actual)	FY 2007 (est.)	FY 2008 (est.)
HSR	873	887	940	929	921	920
Total NIH budget	27,066	27,887	28,495	28,461	28,578	28,858
% HSR in NIH budget	3%	3%	3%	3%	3%	3%

NOTE: HSR = health services research; NIH = National Institutes of Health.

focused on health services research such as community person-nel, economic issues, and utilization. Research on quality is only a minority of submitted applications, Kramer said.

Health services researchers may apply to numerous agencies; this discussion focused specifically on applications to either the NIH or AHRQ. Research proposals may be divided among agencies in a variety of ways. Applications may be "preassigned," where either AHRQ or the NIH is requested by an investigator. Applications may also be "reviewed and referred," a method in which a division within the NIH assigns applications to either agency. Finally, every application for more than $300,000 in the area of health services research is automatically sent to the NIH, Kramer explained.

DISCUSSION

Research Budget

Clancy explained that resources in AHRQ's budget for grant applications outside priority areas (e.g., patient safety, health infor-mation technology, care management/prevention, and comparative effectiveness) are severely limited; applications for the priority areas are capped at $300,000 (total cost) per year. Additionally, there are clear expectations that much of AHRQ's budget should be invested in key areas such as patient safety and information technology.

In response to a question about why the NIH's health services research funding has stayed relatively flat, Kramer said that although 3 percent of the NIH budget (equating to approximately $920 mil-lion) is a substantial amount of money, about 80 percent of grants are awarded to investigator-initiated awards. Kramer viewed the steady percentage of funding, especially in a time of budget restraints, as a sign of hope for quality improvement research.

A question was asked about whether either agency would conduct the same activities it does now if its budget was 3 times greater or if there were specific areas in which further investments would be made. Although current resources cannot fund certain areas, Clancy said, more needs to be done than continuously collecting examples of great work. Clancy would invest in information technology networks, finding ways to allow information technology infrastructures to be reused. Another area needing attention is the extension of efforts to include vulnerable populations and institutions. Kramer noted that the NIH constantly thinks of expansion, citing the NIH Roadmap, which identified underfunded, crosscutting areas to help achieve the NIH mission. One idea from the Roadmap was the Clinical Translational Science Awards, which are granted to networks of interlocking academic health centers focused on translational science.

Funders' Roles in Research

Clancy posed the question of whether funders of health care services should support the development of quality measures because such support potentially could be viewed as a conflict of interest. Agencies such as the Centers for Medicare & Medicaid Services are currently involved in both roles; it is unclear what the relationship should be because it has been shown to have both positive and negative consequences. The right place for this nexus between researchers and policy makers should be discussed, said Raynard Kington of the NIH.

In response to a question about what roles the NIH and AHRQ should play in prioritizing research and the criteria for doing so, Clancy noted that resources in quality improvement should be prioritized with public input. Money should be invested where the biggest problems are. Only 10 percent or less should focus on emerging challenges and innovations. Kramer agreed, adding that there must be a compromise; it is unclear where the line should be drawn because both play a role. Prioritization should not be simply top down.

Transparency

The recent focus on transparency has been both a hindrance and an ally, Clancy said. It has been a hindrance because it promotes thinking that quality improvement and implementation are not sciences. Transparency has been an ally in that it helps people understand what health care managers are confronting on a daily basis. However, without science, managers do not know where to start or which interventions to employ to improve quality. Good theories and frameworks to unify concepts in ways that fit together are missing. Although significant advances have been made, much more needs to be done. O'Neill noted that the focus should not be on management, but rather on leadership.

Data Collection

O'Neill cited a recent study that found that 47 percent of children do not receive medically indicated care (Mangione-Smith et al., 2007). This research, based on medical records, begs the questions of whether medical records are legitimate bases for generalized results and whether research findings need follow-up. In response, Kramer noted that data from medical records do indeed limit research because they only approximate what actually occurred. However, these records are critical to quality improvement research and health services research, which are dominated by retrospective looks at charts and medical records. Fields are always enhanced if prospectively collected information can be interjected, Kramer said. Clancy stated that what this says about the field of research is that knowledge—not application—is prized.

Answering a question about initiatives for the secondary use of data, Clancy noted that partnerships with integrated delivery systems and physician practice networks have been developing, although common data definitions are still needed, both for research and for quality improvement.

Relationship Between Quality Improvement and Research

One audience member said his impression from the panel was that quality improvement has been divorced from research. If the purpose is to improve health, quality improvement research and clinical research could be viewed as a continuum, with quality improvement research conducted before clinical research begins. If so, should health care delivery research design trials to answer questions important to advancing biology? Kramer responded that the times and contexts in which health care is practiced are changing and that therefore quality improvement should also be changing. One impediment is the belief among individual physicians that clinical judgment dominates. The notion that the two have been "divorced" is a depiction of perspectives from 10 to 20 years ago. Kramer now believes the fields are moving in the right direction, albeit slowly.

Another person asked about the relationship between cost-effectiveness and quality of life. Kramer responded that the two are separate but connected. Although quality of life remains difficult to capture, increasing attention is being paid to quality of life and more economists and quality-of-life experts are being incorporated into study teams.

The IOM Forum on the Science of Health Care Quality Improvement and Implementation should focus on the urgent need to build a science base for quality improvement, said Clancy, in response to a question about what this group can do to really change health care.

3

Research as a Driving
Force for Change

"Never doubt that a small group of thoughtful committed people can change the world; indeed it's the only thing that ever has!"

—Meade

There is an increasing challenge to translate and disseminate evaluation results in such a manner that they may be used in decision-making processes to improve health and health care, said Lori Melichar of the Robert Wood Johnson Foundation. To address the state of quality improvement research and its role in improving the health care system, panelists discussed the roles of foundations and academia in research, providing a sense for how research should be used to inform decision making and create the business case. Panelists were asked to discuss the following questions:

- Are there effective research-oriented models in practice aimed at the translation of outcomes from improvement research to effective operational practices?
- What are the relevant direct research capabilities and infrastructure support required to build and sustain this research, and what are the current and future extramural funding sources that will share the investment costs with institutions?
- What measurements are relevant to evaluate the return on this investment and future sustainability of quality improvement research?
- Can a priority agenda for quality improvement research be identified nationally to stimulate and validate such research efforts?

OVERVIEW

Jeffrey Alexander of the University of Michigan opened the session, offering high-level impressions of the state of quality improvement research and suggesting changes likely to make quality improvement research more relevant, useful, and practical to decision makers.

Beginning with his perspective on quality improvement research, Alexander noted that many studies are performed in single organizations (e.g., large university teaching hospitals), which raises questions about whether the interventions would be effective in community hospitals, small inner-city hospitals, or other institutions. Second, the literature indicates that research tends to be opportunistic rather than systematic. Research is often conducted by faculty members at large teaching hospitals who see opportunities for testing interventions, such as process changes that have been introduced by administrative or clinical leaders in their organizations. However, research should be conducted in a more planned, systematic manner. Third, quality improvement research often suffers from imprecise measurement and description of the quality improvement intervention, which limits adoption of the intervention by other organizations or replication of the research by others. In contrast to the way clinical research is advanced (i.e., replication of trials with different samples in different settings), little replication exists in quality improvement research. Fourth, most studies are of relatively short duration, often lasting 12 to 18 months or less, precluding conclusions from being drawn about sustainability of changes. Fifth, there are often no explicit considerations of the organizational contexts or factors affecting implementation of an intervention. Sixth, explicit considerations of cost or value are often lacking.

As a result of these six problems with the quality improvement literature, Alexander concluded there is inconsistent information regarding what works, when it works, where it works, and what it costs. An opportunity therefore exists to rethink how quality improvement research could be conducted to become more valid, generalizable, and useful to decision makers.

To act on the opportunity for quality improvement, Alexander looked toward policy, informational, and financial barriers to quality improvement. The reimbursement system does not pay for quality, despite the Centers for Medicare & Medicaid Services' (CMS') recent efforts to not pay for preventable errors and pay for performance. The tipping point has not yet been reached where these programs will make large differences in care, Alexander said. From the perspective of consumers, information is still not readily available to help patients distinguish between good and poor quality care. Further, the information that is available has not been shown to have influenced patients' decision making, Alexander said. Additionally, little consideration has been given by major funding agencies to study implementation of quality improvement practices.

The traditional, linear model of basic research to the deployment of a treatment is not working, as evidenced by the insufficient uptake of organizations adopting best practices. A new model is needed that would take into consideration implementation as a component of quality improvement research and the effects of contextual factors on implementation and quality improvement effectiveness. Although implementation research is not yet at a point that it can be called implementation science, Alexander noted, it is clear that factors affecting implementation can be divided into categories such as process, content, internal context, and external context. However, how these issues work together to predict and design effective implementation strategies remains unclear. Distinctions are often made among adoption, implementation, diffusion, and institutionalization or sustainability, Alexander added. While considerable research exists about adoption, relatively little exists about implementation, and almost none exists about perhaps the most important pieces: diffusion and institutionalization within and across organizations.

To develop the capacity to strengthen quality improvement research, Alexander offered five suggestions. First, funding must be increased and more nonrandomized controlled trials should be supported. Second, multidisciplinary teams should be used more broadly because research is currently being conducted mostly by physicians, not economists or organizational researchers. Third, implementation should be considered part of the intervention, not as a by-product. Fourth, the duration of studies should be lengthened in order to draw conclusions about sustainability of an intervention. Finally, cost-effectiveness should be incorporated into the research agenda.

EXAMPLES OF QUALITY IMPROVEMENT RESEARCH

Patrick Romano of the University of California, Davis, presented two examples for quality improvement research, offering lessons learned from each to improve both the validity and the interpretation of research.

Computerized provider order entry (CPOE) systems were found

to reduce serious medication errors by 60 percent in one major teaching hospital (Bates et al., 1999). As a result, a substantial movement toward adopting these systems began; in particular, efforts spearheaded by the Leapfrog Group gained attention.[1] Although these findings were persuasive, Romano said, a significant decrease in adverse drug events was not demonstrated. Recently, questions have been raised about these findings. First, a qualitative study identified 22 different types of errors facilitated by CPOE systems (e.g., separation of functions resulting in double dosing and incompatible orders; system crashes delaying medication orders; automatic cancellation of medications after surgery), some of which resulted inadvertently in harm (Koppel et al., 2005). Another study described unintended adverse consequences of CPOE systems, such as errors in communicating and coordinating processes (Ash et al., 2004), while a third study found a dramatic increase in risk-adjusted mortality among children transferred into an academic children's hospital for specialized care, as a result of implementation problems (Han et al., 2005). Several of these single-system studies showed conflicting results, largely because of heterogeneity in how CPOE is implemented. Although pressure for widespread adoption exists, more time may be needed to fully assess the evidence. More harm than good may have resulted from the implementation of CPOE systems in some settings, but there is no way of knowing because no ongoing system for monitoring the nationwide impact exists, Romano said.

The second example Romano presented was about one of the Joint Commission's core measures of hospital quality: time to first antibiotic dose within 4 hours of admission for community-acquired pneumonia. This indicator, supported and endorsed by CMS and the National Quality Forum, is based on evidence from observational studies of thousands of patients, showing 15 percent reductions in both in-hospital and 30-day mortality with prompt administration of antibiotics. However, the evidence has limitations: The exact time period was never well established (no significant difference was found between 4 and 8 hours), and mortality did not decrease for those with prior antibiotic treatment. Recently, concerns about the measure's validity arose. Due to the 4-hour imperative, 20 percent of patients treated according to this measure at one center left the emergency department without a diagnosis of pneumonia. Another

---

[1]The Leapfrog Group is sponsored by the Business Roundtable to improve health care quality. One of its main "leaps" forward to improve patient safety is to encourage widespread implementation of CPOE systems.

study showed that delayed antibiotic therapy in the emergency department is often due to legitimate diagnostic uncertainty or heavy patient load, highlighting the need for adequate systems of care outside the hospital. Finally, researchers discovered that since the measure's introduction, pneumonia has been overdiagnosed. At one teaching hospital, 30 percent of patients admitted with a presumptive diagnosis of pneumonia are now discharged with a noninfectious diagnosis. The consequences of such overdiagnosis remain unclear, Romano said.

Many lessons can be learned from these examples. Most importantly, quality improvement interventions differ fundamentally from prescription drugs in that they are inherently heterogeneous. CPOE systems all differ, while the same system likely varies between hospitals. As a result, implementation and context make huge differences, Romano concluded. Premature acceptance of new interventions based on surrogate markers is a real and serious issue, as described in the previous examples. Unintended consequences must be considered before widespread implementation occurs. Surveillance systems should be established to facilitate ongoing monitoring of these unintended consequences when new information technologies are introduced.

Specifically addressing quality improvement research, problems of internal and external validity may arise, Romano said. Although threats to internal validity do not necessarily affect all studies, they can be avoided through clever study designs. These threats include confounding, information bias, and patient selection and attrition biases. Threats to external validity include generalizability to other regions, settings, and facilities, as well as publication bias. To face these threats, Romano suggested that a number of research methods could be employed. Cluster randomization is the best method for evaluating quality improvement interventions that are implemented at the hospital or clinic level. Recognizing the need for concurrent control or comparison groups, quasi-experimental study designs could be used to minimize confounding and improve internal validity. Interrupted time series analyses are another approach to isolating the effect of an intervention. One key challenge is to create data systems that would allow evaluators to easily and efficiently find control variables. To minimize other biases, researchers should be blinded, implementation *processes* should be measured, and long-term outcomes should be evaluated in addition to short-term outcomes.

Infrastructure should be enhanced to allow quality improvement research to advance health care. To improve generalizability, studies should involve multiple institutions from a variety of regions and practice types. Data systems and registries must be supported to facilitate ongoing evaluations of the impact of interventions, Romano said. This expanded infrastructure for quality improvement research will enable more cross-institutional studies, multidisciplinary studies, researcher training, and funding, which are also necessary to improve the infrastructure. Conceptual frameworks from the social sciences and analytic methods from biostatistics and econometrics are examples of what should be borrowed and adapted from other disciplines. With respect to training, organizations such as the Department of Veterans Affairs (VA), the Agency for Healthcare Research and Quality, and the Health Resources and Services Administration fund programs in this area, but there has been little systematic effort to bring nonphysicians into the field.

With respect to funding, the current investment in research and evaluation is inadequate. State and local governments should recognize that they have large stakes in health care quality and should become more involved in applied quality improvement research, leveraging programs such as Medicaid and worker's compensation. Another point of examination should be the payment system because those people investing resources to improve quality tend not to be the actual recipients of financial rewards. To supplement current efforts, quality improvement should be linked to the National Institutes of Health's Clinical and Translational Science Awards program and focus on translating science from the clinical level to the population or community level.

DEPARTMENT OF VETERANS AFFAIRS INITIATIVES

The VA has been a leader in improving quality, said Joel Kupersmith of the VA. With an annual budget of $35 billion, 5.5 million patients, and more than 1,400 sites of care, the VA has implemented a wide variety of efforts to improve care delivery, such as adoption of evidence-based practice guidelines, quality measures, leadership, and an electronic health record system (which, Kupersmith noted, was a bottom-up development by individual academic physicians). The VA also developed the Quality Enhancement Research Initiative (QUERI) to make evidence-based practices part of routine clinical practice, resulting in fundamental cultural change. Cultural change should trump technological change every time, Kupersmith said. To facilitate this, QUERI promotes research with continuous evaluation, usually of disease-specific processes. QUERI also develops and implements strategies for change, implemented first in single-site pilots and eventually implemented systemwide.

Giving two examples of quality improvement research at the VA, Kupersmith first introduced the administration's work in schizophrenia. Schizophrenia effects 1 percent of people, about 100,000 VA patients a year. Although this number is less than 2 percent of VA patients, care for people with schizophrenia equates to a much larger percentage of the VA's health care costs. It had been shown that outcomes can improve with an evidence-based approach (e.g., appropriate medications, caregiver involvement, vocational rehabilitation), but many schizophrenics do not receive proper care. The purpose of the VA's program was to identify gaps between evidence and practice. By performing formative and summative research assessments, measures of evidence-based prescribing and side-effect management both improved for schizophrenia. Medication noncompliance was not significantly impacted. However, the success of the program led to the realization that management and improvement in treatment of schizophrenia are possible. As a result, a second program began, based on the formative evaluations of the study.

Offering a second example, Kupersmith said patients with spinal cord injuries were observed to have high mortality rates from respiratory disorders. A random survey of patient characteristics showed that patients with specific characteristics such as being older and nonsmokers got their vaccines, but others did not. However, the findings were only validated by modifying the study's protocol during the study (e.g., more broadly targeting veterans, including more disorders, increasing the use of standing orders).

Different approaches in basic, clinical, and organizational research will be required to fully study the implementation of quality improvement interventions. Researchers do not often view quality improvement research as true hard-core research, Kupersmith said, while chief executive officers do not necessarily consider it organizational. The field is more qualitative, with different end points and a different vocabulary. This research is observational and interventional, formative as well as summative. The VA has successfully advanced the quality-of-care agenda by leveraging the administrative system, the electronic health record, and high-quality research capabilities. Substantial improvement requires organizational and cultural changes, which are difficult to achieve.

DISCUSSION

Generalizability

In response to a question about generalizability, Kupersmith noted that it is harder to translate efforts outside the VA than within the VA because it is a system with specific attributes. Translating efforts within the VA is not entirely possible because patients are all different.

The challenge is to learn how to be vigilant within one's own institution and learn how to share lessons with others without fear of liability or embarrassment, Romano said. Groups must share what they have learned and publish that information so others can benefit. Using the pneumonia example, must people be needlessly scared about getting unnecessary antibiotics in order for others who need the antibiotics to get them on time? Health care should learn from other industries that also encounter the need to reduce errors, such as the airline industry, where the costs associated with having error-free systems are built into business models. These trade-offs are beginning to be identified, but must be made explicit. Kupersmith agreed, stating that transparency is critical for any quality improvement effort or research.

Culture

Alexander suggested two truisms of culture. First, changing culture in a small organization is different from in large, complex organizations. This is partly because large organizations do not have one culture, but multiple subcultures. Instead, a superordinate culture should be created that embraces the subcultures. This task is different from changing culture within a small hospital. Second, physician groups face less of a culture issue but more of an organizational climate issue. These groups often practice with a "siege mentality" and do not want to look outside of what is currently available, given the other pressures they are experiencing. A lot of work is involved to change behaviors in these organizations, Alexander concluded.

4

Breakout Groups

Workshop attendees were asked to split into three breakout groups, each discussing one of the following: defining the value proposition, effective intraorganizational spread of quality improvement gains, and effective industrywide quality improvement gains.

VALUE PROPOSITION

The value proposition is a plan that will enhance value for patients by improving outcomes, lowering costs, or both, said Laura Leviton of the Robert Wood Johnson Foundation, reporting for the value proposition group. Discussion of this working definition led to the realization that there were actually two different value propositions in question: one for quality improvement itself and one for research on quality improvement.

The value proposition for quality improvement must take into account three different perspectives, Leviton said. First, the patient must be the focus of all interventions, at a reasonable cost. Second, while alignment of all interests is praiseworthy, it must be acknowledged that quality improvement will most likely not be a win–win situation for everyone. In the end, the value proposition must focus on what is best for society and individual patients. Recognizing the second perspective, the group identified a third perspective: There should be research to study the value proposition. While the goal is to promote having informed patients, the challenge remains doing so effectively, which requires efforts to promote transparency both in terms of costs and quality outcomes.

Creating a value proposition for *research* on quality improvement is somewhat different than for quality improvement itself and involves a number of issues. Recognition that data give weight to health care leaders' desire to champion and implement quality improvement was an important point in the discussion. Becoming better at translating the research available for uptake is urgently needed because research is done for a purpose, not merely for its own sake. Priorities for quality improvement research must be set, Leviton said, because they allow society to effectively allocate resources. Having priorities would also help to articulate the potential value of quality improvement, as has occurred successfully with cancer research (number of lives saved) and smoking cessation research (the societal effect of quit rates). Finally, data currently being gathered are not tracking outcomes that matter. Data should be collected over time, which could be facilitated by electronic health records and could have beneficial effects on improving patient education and producing health care reform.

INTRAORGANIZATIONAL QUALITY
IMPROVEMENT GAINS

Effective intraorganizational quality improvement gains must be created within an environment where quality is a top priority and not just a short-term project, O'Neill said, reporting for the breakout group that explored that topic. Organizations successfully improving quality do not have an attitude of "we're great at everything we do," but instead think of ways to continuously improve. Quality improvement and safety should be automatic within an organization to promote change.

A number of common themes arose from this breakout group. First, there is an essential need for transparency, as found in the value proposition group. Management and top leadership must accept responsibility for everything that goes wrong within an organization because doing so gives those people actually making mistakes permission to identify their mistakes. People must not be punished, blamed, or criticized for their mistakes so that lessons can be learned to prevent the same mistakes from recurring.

Second, having clear objectives is critical to make progress both within and across organizations. Clarity of objectives allows people to relate and understand how they need to function in relation to agreed-on goals.

Third, the group identified a need to deal with things gone wrong. People must deal with intraorganizational transfer in a manner as close to real time as possible, allowing for connections to be made between observations and the change and success of new experiments. Everyone within an organization must believe in the ability to improve and the methods for doing so. Those not willing to attempt to improve actually destroy the ability to change for those who want to get it right, O'Neill said. Deviation from producing the right outcomes and perfect care cannot be tolerated. Improvement can only be fostered in a blame-free culture.

INDUSTRYWIDE QUALITY IMPROVEMENT

Richard Kahn of the American Diabetes Association (ADA) recapped the industrywide quality improvement group's discussion, which focused on four examples of widespread interventions and some commonalities.

The first example was administration of beta blockers after an acute myocardial infarction (MI). The first study that showed some benefit of this therapy was published in 1982, but the use of beta blockers did not really gain traction until the mid-1990s, when the American College of Cardiology/American Heart Association developed guidelines recommending the use of the drug after an MI. Around the same time, the National Committee for Quality Assurance and the Joint Commission developed a performance measure for beta blockers, which led to the development of incentives and tools to encourage the use of beta blockers by health plans and others. At the onset of reporting, data showed that approximately 60 percent of people with MIs received beta blockers soon after the event. Recently, this number has grown to more than 90 percent, and because of its success, the measure has been retired.

Smoking cessation counseling was the second example of an industrywide quality improvement intervention. After the first surgeon general's report on smoking cessation, states and the federal government became involved, and the public's concern grew. It was later found that physicians had an influence on smoking cessation rates. A performance measure was then developed for physicians to initiate discussions about counseling. Smoking cessation counseling now occurs nearly 100 percent of the time, and the health care industry along with other forces can take credit for reducing the prevalence of smoking, Kahn stated.

Testing hemoglobin A1c (HbA1c) levels can determine glycemic control in people with diabetes. This is an essential test for guiding treatment and establishing treatment goals. In the early 1980s the first report appeared, indicating that the amount of glucose bound to hemoglobin was a good surrogate measure of the circulating glucose concentrations over the preceding 3 to 4 months. In 1993 the first well-controlled study was published showing that HbA1c was an excellent predictor of diabetes complications, and any reduction in HbA1c would reduce the likelihood of complications. In 1995 a performance measure for HbA1c was developed (patients with diabetes should receive at least one HbA1c measurement annually). A variety of tools were developed by the ADA and the National Diabetes Education Program to help promote the use of the HbA1c test and to use the HbA1c level as a treatment target. Performance improved (i.e., number of patients receiving at least one test annually) from around 60 percent in the mid-1990s to a current level of about 97 percent.

The final example provided was childhood vaccinations. Changes in law and public policy played a large role in vaccination rates when schools required all children to be vaccinated. State and county governments provided financial support for vaccines to be distributed to physicians or schools.

These four examples shared three common themes, Kahn said. First, they were all discrete and focused interventions. Second, the intervention and the desired outcome were closely linked. Third, guidelines and performance measures were developed by credible organizations. Nonetheless, how individual institutions actually implemented these interventions remains unclear because no literature has documented the exact steps or determined the most effective and efficient methods of implementation. Much like teaching a child to ride a bike, there is no exact science or literature that describes the best, most efficient learning process, but widespread success is eventually achieved.

5

Communicating a Value Proposition

A major barrier to improving quality is the receptivity of the management and leadership of health care institutions, Thomas Boat said.

INTEGRATING THE BUSINESS LANGUAGE

For quality improvement to have its next big impact, it must be brought to the level of chief executive officers (CEOs) and chief financial officers (CFOs), Scott Hamlin said. Hamlin offered that the concepts articulated during the workshop were the correct ones, but the next step is to incorporate the language of business into researchers' and policy makers' thinking. Without embracing the language of CEOs and CFOs, they can never be brought along to understand what needs to be done. CEOs and CFOs are the ones who influence boards, shareholders, and trustees' decisions, and they are responsible for the delivery of value. Boards, shareholders, and payers all share one common language—market share.

To integrate the business language, competitive advantage must be addressed because it is the CEO's and CFO's primary concern. Hamlin described competitive advantage as specific characteristics of the organization that are marketable and that positively differentiate the organization from others. Researchers and policy makers must help decision makers understand how quality improvement and quality improvement research translate into competitive advantages. The disconnect Hamlin saw between the workshop discussions and where the discussions needed to be to capture the attention of leadership was the business model. In defining a business model, a business case is usually made, followed by case examples supporting it. In health care, the opposite seems to happen. Case studies are often used as proof of a business case, but are rarely presented in the context of the entity's articulated business model or business strategy. Hamlin provided the following business model as an example: Cincinnati Children's Hospital Medical Center is located in a small metropolitan area and relies on a substantial portion of its inpatient revenues to come from patients traveling from outside its primary service area; many patients must bypass multiple other options along the way. To justify patients' efforts, or the trust of a referring physician, the Cincinnati Children's Hospital Medical Center must have a demonstrable outcome advantage or provide a cost advantage for a comparable outcome. This is the business model and shows the importance of quality. Improved quality carries the ammunition to attack both sides of the "value equation": product differentiation from better outcomes and/or lower costs.

As an academically affiliated organization, Cincinnati Children's Hospital Medical Center's care is suboptimal because no patient stays in a division or department throughout an entire inpatient stay. This is one of the biggest challenges to optimizing value, Hamlin said, noting that although academic structures can inhibit quality improvement, the highly successful pieces must be built up. The CEO's and CFO's roles are to help each line be as successful as possible. If parts of the system are suboptimal, they must work together to find a solution, not just focus on the specialties in which they are competitive. The problem is not the reimbursement system, Hamlin said, because people will always find ways to maximize profits in reimbursement systems. The real key is to improve the quality, and thereby the value, of health care.

THE NEED FOR RESEARCH

Research partnerships with clinical care are imperative. The research and development arm of a health care institution cannot be a separate group and must be engaged in the decision-making process, Hamlin said. Examples of success, such as those described during the first panel, can influence others to improve the quality of care they provide, Boat said. Although successful spread can occur in this manner, it will not be entirely successful without an evidence base to convince an organization's leadership that it can improve health outcomes and ultimately lower costs.

A balance must be struck between generating evidence to support improvement efforts and convincing institutions to implement indicated changes, Boat recommended, adding that every quality improvement effort should include an analytic component. Before each intervention, the intervener and data analyst must know what data to collect, how to collect them, and how to analyze them. The best and most appropriate analytic tools available should be used to study each intervention because randomized controlled trials are not always the best approach. The best analytic techniques should be applied to better evaluate the potential impacts of interventions.

Predictive modeling of interventions is another role for research, Boat said. The best evidence available should be used to identify health care risks and plan interventions that avoid those risks. Reacting to and reducing adverse events and waste in medical care must happen in real time. For this purpose, investigators should work with clinicians and hospital management to facilitate decision-making processes.

OTHER AUDIENCES AND AREAS

During this discussion, other areas for the forum to pursue arose and are summarized below.

Adherence

The lack of patient adherence to prescribed care prevents medicine from being as effective as it could be, Boat said. Although there are data documenting that 50 percent of people do not receive indicated care, approximately 50 percent of care also is never delivered because of lack of adherent patient behaviors. This stems from inadequate partnering for health care planning with the true caregivers, the patients themselves and their families. There is a need for these caregivers to understand how to manage their health care; without this component, quality of care does not matter, Boat said. The forum should address the issue of adherence and self-management in the future because health care is really about self-care.

Equity

Issues of equity, especially regarding the underinsured or those with mixed copays, are challenging when developing a business case, Marshall Chin said. Hamlin agreed that this was a daunting issue, but said that if quality is not resolved first, equity cannot be addressed. Equity is not the main issue; poor utilization of resources is.

Organizational Theory

Organizational theory is a field from which quality improvement should learn, O'Neill said, referencing the field's contributions to other industries. Organizational theorists could inform health care about the types of organizations that are more or less likely to succeed in the objective delivery of health care. Of particular use would be organizational structure, hierarchy, and leadership models.

References

Ash, J. S., M. Berg, and E. Coiera. 2004. Some unintended consequences of information technology in health care: The nature of patient care information system-related errors. *Journal of the American Medical Informatics Association* 11(2):104-112.

Bates, D. W., J. M. Teich, J. Lee, D. Seger, G. J. Kuperman, N. Ma'Luf, D. Boyle, and L. Leape. 1999. The impact of computerized physician order entry on medication error prevention. *Journal of the American Medical Informatics Association* 6(4):313-321.

Han, Y. Y., J. A. Carcillo, S. T. Venkataraman, R. S. B. Clark, R. S. Watson, T. C. Nguyen, H. Bayir, and R. A. Orr. 2005. Unexpected increased mortality after implementation of a commercially sold computerized physician order entry system. *Pediatrics* 116(6):1506-1512.

Koppel, R., J. P. Metlay, A. Cohen, B. Abaluck, A. R. Localio, S. E. Kimmel, and B. L. Strom. 2005. Role of computerized physician order entry systems in facilitating medication errors. *Journal of the American Medical Association* 293(10):1197-1203.

Leatherman, S., D. Berwick, D. Iles, L. S. Lewin, F. Davidoff, T. Nolan, and M. Bisognano. 2003. The business case for quality: Case studies and an analysis. *Health Affairs* 22(2):17-30.

Mangione-Smith, R., A. H. DeCristofaro, C. M. Setodji, J. Keesey, D. J. Klein, J. L. Adams, M. A. Schuster, and E. A. McGlynn. 2007. The quality of ambulatory care delivered to children in the United States. *New England Journal of Medicine* 357(15):1515-1523.

McCauley, K. M., M. B. Bixby, and M. D. Naylor. 2006. Advanced practice nurse strategies to improve outcomes and reduce cost in elders with heart failure. *Disease Management* 9(5):302-310.

Naylor, M. D., D. A. Brooten, R. L. Campbell, G. Maislin, K. M. McCauley, and J. S. Schwartz. 2004. Transitional care of older adults hospitalized with heart failure: A randomized, controlled trial. *Journal of the American Geriatrics Society* 52(5):675-684.

Titler, M., J. Dochterman, D. M. Picone, L. Everett, X. J. Xie, M. Kanak, and Q. Fei. 2005. Cost of hospital care for elderly at risk of falling. *Nursing Economics* 23(6):290-306.

Appendix A

Workshop Agenda

Creating a Business Case for Quality Improvement and
Quality Improvement Research

Monday, October 15, 2007
Doubletree Hotel
Crystal City, VA
8:30 am–5:30 pm

8:30 am   **Welcome and Overview of Workshop, Including Objectives and Goals**
Thomas Boat, Forum Co-Chair
Paul O'Neill, Forum Co-Chair
Scott Hamlin, Planning Committee Leader

9:00 am   **Session 1: The Business Case for Quality and Quality Improvement Research**
Herb Fritch, HealthSpring
James Bagian, Department of Veterans Affairs
Steve Spear, Massachusetts Institute of Technology
    and Institute for Healthcare Improvement
Gary Kaplan, Virginia Mason
Marita Titler, University of Iowa

Moderator: Paul O'Neill, Forum Co-Chair
- Issues to Be Addressed:
  o Is there a business case in today's health care environment that is responsive and relevant to the leadership of health care and related research enterprises (including providers, payers, patients, government officials, academia, and employers)?
  o Is so, what are the economic/financial benefits of pursuing quality improvements and related

research in the field? Illustrate how quality improvement and quality improvement research can impact greater production use of plant and human assets, lead to product differentiation and branding, generate revenue enhancements, improve cost structure, and impact other core operational goals to create competitive advantages.

o What are the characteristics of an ideal enterprise culture and effective governance orientation that promote and accelerate improvement in quality and quality improvement research?

o What are the business disciplines and support structures that are essential for leadership to fully exploit the economic/financial benefits of quality improvement and quality improvement research?

o In order to drive organizational improvement from validated, well-researched data, how do you effectively measure and evaluate progress against quality improvement targets and quantify returns on investments made? What are the essential components of such a system?

o Are there models in other industries such as aviation and nuclear power wherein the drive for quality has transformed product outcomes and customer/public safety? How do we learn from them?

11:30 am   **Working Lunch**

12:30 pm   **Session 2: The Role of Policy Makers**
Carolyn Clancy, Agency for Healthcare Research and
      Quality
Barnett S. Kramer, National Institutes of Health

Moderator: Denise Cardo, Centers for Disease
      Control and Prevention
  • Issues to Be Addressed:
    o What are the fundamental public policy features and objectives that will lead to a transformational improvement in the quality and economic viability of our health care system?

> o What role does transparency of outcomes and cost data play in driving quality improvement? How can quality improvement research better support these efforts? What public policy features might help to unleash its potential?
> o What public policy features are essential to help finance, promote, and reward relevant research into quality improvement sciences?

1:50 pm   **Break**

2:00 pm   **Session 3: Research as a Driving Force for Quality Improvement and Broad Implementation**
Jeffrey Alexander, University of Michigan
Patrick Romano, University of California, Davis
Joel Kupersmith, Department of Veterans Affairs

Moderator: Lori Melichar, The Robert Wood Johnson Foundation
- Issues to Be Addressed:
  - o Are there effective research-oriented models in practice aimed at the translation of outcomes from improvement research to effective operational practices?
  - o What are the relevant direct research capabilities and infrastructure support required to build and sustain this research, and what are the current and future extramural funding sources that will share the investment costs with institutions?
  - o What measurements are relevant to evaluate the return on this investment and future sustainability of quality improvement research?
  - o Can a priority agenda for quality improvement research be identified nationally to stimulate and validate such research efforts?

3:20 pm   **Breakout Groups**
- Group 1 Topic Discussion—Developing the value proposition statement
- Group 2 Topic Discussion—Effective intraorganizational spread of quality improvement gains
- Group 3 Topic Discussion—Effective industrywide spread of quality improvement gains

4:20 pm   **Reports Back to Group**

4:45 pm   **Wrap-Up Session: Creating and Communicating a
                 Value Proposition**

                 Moderator: Thomas Boat, Forum Co-Chair
           •   Issues to Be Addressed:
                 o Who generates the value proposition statement
                    and who is the targeted audience?
                 o What are the targeted venues of communication?
                 o Other "next steps" to move forward?

5:30 pm   **Adjourn**

Appendix B

Workshop Participants

Karen Adams
National Quality Forum

Bradley Beauvais
U.S. Army–Baylor Graduate
    Program

Bona Benjamin
American Society of Health-
    System Pharmacists

Bernice Bennett
National Association of Public
    Hospitals and Health
    Systems

Erica Breslau
National Cancer Institute

Maureen Broms
New England Baptist Hospital

Denise Cardo[*]
Centers for Disease Control and
    Prevention

Andrew Cohen
AGC & Associates

Patrick Conway
White House Fellow, Agency
    for Healthcare Research
    and Quality

Louis Diamond
Thomson Healthcare

Molla Donaldson
George Washington University
    School of Medicine and
    Health Services

Denise Dougherty[*]
Agency for Healthcare Research
    and Quality

---

[*]Representative for ex-officio members.

Michael Ellwood
American Academy of
    Physicians Assistants

Gary Filerman
Georgetown University

Angela Franklin
American College of Emergency
    Physicians

Linda Greenberg
Agency for Healthcare Research
    and Quality

Rachel Groman
American Association of
    Neurosurgery/CNS

Jenissa Haidari
American Academy of
    Otolaryngology

Allison Hamblin
Center for Health Care
    Strategies, Inc.

Bruce Hamory
Geisinger Health System

Janet Heinrich
Health Policy R&D

Mary Johnston
Accreditation Council for
    Graduate Medical
    Education

Stephanie Jones
American Academy of
    Otolaryngology–Head and
    Neck Surgery

Beth Kosiak
American Urological
    Association

Russ Mardon
OMRG

Ronald McDade
MedStar Health

Linda McKibben
The McKibben Group

David Meyers
EmCare, Inc.

Rachel Nelson
Centers for Medicare &
    Medicaid Services

Karen Pennar
Hudson Health Plan

Hoangmai Pham
Center for Studying Health
    System Change

Peter Pronovost
Johns Hopkins University
    School of Medicine

Siddharta Reddy
American Board of Internal
    Medicine

Susan Rossi[*]
National Institutes of Health

Cynthia Saunders
Maryland Health Services Cost
    Review Commission

Pamela Scarrow
American College of
Obstetricians and
Gynecologists

Mark Smith
Department of Veterans Affairs,
Palo Alto

Vivian Speer
Remedy MD

Lisa Sprague
George Washington University

David Stevens
Agency for Healthcare Research
and Quality

Robin Stombler
Auburn Health Strategies, LLC

Janet (Jessie) Sullivan
Hudson Health Plan

Kasey Thompson
American Society of Health-
System Pharmacists